THE HOT TUB DIET

GET OUT OF THE GYM
INTO THE HOT TUB
AND LOSE WEIGHT

BY
BRIDGET PRAYTOR

THE HOT TUB DIET. Copyright © 2012

Library of Congress Cataloging-in-Publication Data

Bridget Praytor
The Hot Tub Diet
ISBN -13: 978-1477446119

Cover Photo by ©Depositphotos/Antony McAulay

All information provided in The Hot Tub Diet is for information purposes only. The Hot Tub Diet Book may contain information that is created and maintained by a variety of sources both external and internal. In no event shall the author of The Hot Tub Diet be responsible or liable, directly or indirectly, for any damage or loss caused or alleged to be caused by or in connection with the use of or reliance on any information found in the book. Health related topics found in The Hot Tub Diet, should not be used for diagnosing purposes or be substituted for medical advice. As with any new or ongoing treatment, always consult your professional healthcare providers before beginning any new treatment. It is your responsibility to research the accuracy, completeness, and usefulness of all found information provided in this book, including the information found on external resources. It is your responsibility to consult with your general practitioner whether such information can benefit you in any way. The author of The Hot Tub Diet assumes no responsibility or liability for any consequence resulting directly or indirectly for any action or inaction you take based on or made in reliance on the information, services, or material in this book. The author does not warrant that the information in this book is up to date, complete, true, accurate and non-misleading. The author of The Hot Tub Diet makes no representations or warranties in relation to The Hot Tub Diet book.

DEDICATION

This book is dedicated to everyone that has ever felt overweight or disappointed with the way they look.

ACKNOWLEDGEMENTS

Thank you to my amazing kids who went to bed on time so I could write. Thank you to all my friends and family who have given me encouragement when I have told them the crazy things I wanted to do in life.

TABLE OF CONTENTS

INTRODUCTION

This is not another How-To-Diet or How-To-Exercise book. If anything, it's a How-Not-To-Diet book. Or Stay Sane book. Or Stop Punishing Yourself book. It's a book about how I transformed my life.

Changes in my thinking patterns helped me realize and put into perspective how my weight affected my overall happiness. Mindset changes helped me shed the unwanted pounds. Using the ideas in this book, for the first time in my life I have a body I'm happy with.

For years I knew the "secret" to losing weight that *everyone* knows: eat less and exercise more. But if everyone knows it, why are so many people overweight? It turns out the "secret" is true—but not simple. (If it were simple, all of us would be running out to the mall, excited to go swimsuit shopping.) There is so much more to losing weight. Some people say the "more" is lifestyle, but I disagree. The "more" is mindset.

In the old days I used to think if the scale hit a certain number, my life would be perfect. I was obsessed with how my body looked and I was controlled by food. I used to compare my body to the bodies of models and never be content. Not only did this way of thinking prevent me from losing weight, but it also limited opportunities in my life. After I started to change my mindset, however, I started experiencing major changes in the way I felt about my body and the way my clothes fit. Now I feel great about my body and can look in the mirror and smile. I can also laugh about the areas I have learned to accept. Best of all, I now just care about the way I feel about my body, instead of worrying about what other people think.

I'm writing this book because I've come to realize that my past ways of thinking are common for people who are overweight. I want to share what I've learned and let those people know that their ways of thinking are preventing them from losing weight. By being completely open about my own experiences and how I changed my thought process, I also hope to inspire people who are struggling with their weight. If this book changes one person's life, all the time I've put into writing it will have been worth it.

I've learned to rid myself of ideas that prohibited me from being at a healthy weight. I've stopped looking at myself from a viewpoint that caused me to be constantly discontented. I've learned to focus on the satisfying moments of my life that fill me with happiness. And I also now look great in my jeans.

So where did I discover the secrets to weight loss, true fitness, self-acceptance, and happiness?

Not at the gym or at a weight-loss clinic. Not on one of those TV shows where everyone gets on a scale and publicly confesses to how many calories they consumed that week. Not from one of the thousands of traditional diet books you can buy off the Internet. And not from one of those magazines on the racks in the supermarket checkout lines that promise you a perfect body if you just eat one food—grapefruit, or veal, or broth, or waffles—for an entire month.

I learned it in the hot tub. And so can you.

1

HOT TUB THERAPY

Once upon a time in my life, I was obsessed with exercising. I would spend hours on the treadmill with the other gym rats, going nowhere and accomplishing absolutely nothing. Then I would reward myself something special for working so hard—and when I say special, I mean *special*. Maybe that treat was a huge slice of chocolate cake, or maybe it was "just" a king-size candy bar. Knowing I'd just burned a lot of calories, I would consume this with immense satisfaction. That was my life: exercising a ton, eating whatever I wanted, and rewarding myself constantly because I was always working so hard.

I couldn't understand why the more effort I spent focusing on exercising and "treating" myself right, the more weight I was gaining. And then, in an instant, my life changed.

One minute I was sitting in a parked car at a busy intersection, looking in my rearview mirror and trying to explain to a three- and two-year-old why they needed to only use nice words. The next minute, I was using swear words as I watched a car behind us come up very fast. A moment later, we were rear-ended by it—the driver hadn't realized the light was red.

All I could think about was my children in the back seat. My son was still screaming when the paramedics came rushing to the car. My daughter was in shock, and at first couldn't speak at all. But they calmed down (the paramedic gave them stickers!) and turned out to be uninjured.

I, on the other hand, sustained back and neck injuries. As I lay in the emergency room after a CAT scan, in such extreme pain that I was begging the doctor for more drugs to ease it, he gave me news I thought was devastating: I wouldn't be able to do any strenuous exercise until my back and neck healed.

It baffles me now that I was more upset about *not being able to exercise* than I was about having sustained serious injuries that could have affected me for the rest of my life. But that was how I thought, then.

It would take six months of doctor visits, physical therapy, and chiropractic adjustments for me to finally feel well enough to again be able to exercise strenuously. During those six months, however, I continued to go to the gym to which I'd belonged for years. It offered two free hours of childcare, salvation for a mother of three children under the age of four. Since I couldn't exercise, the only thing I could do there was sit in the hot tub. And so I sat. And talked to people. And listened.

"I'm so fat," I would hear people tell each other as they slipped off towels and got into the water quickly, ashamed of their bodies.

One woman I spoke with looked absolutely gorgeous, but she couldn't stop complaining about her stomach rolls. She talked about how many hours she wasted doing core work, and how no matter what she did the rolls remained. You don't tell a stranger that maybe if she sat up tall and proud, rather than hunched over, those rolls would disappear. But I was thinking it.

Another woman complained about having a hard time losing her "muffin top." I wanted to tell her that maybe she could buy jeans with a slightly higher rise, so they wouldn't accentuate the part of her body she didn't like. Maybe in the right jeans she would stop focusing on how ugly she felt and start realizing how cute she was.

I met an incredibly hot, muscular man who had a body that could have been featured in a fitness magazine. He was incredibly focused on pinching his body fat. How he could find any fat to pinch on that body I still do not know.

Over those six months of sitting in the hot tub I talked to men, women, and teenagers about diets, nutrition, exercise plans, and why "nothing worked." I heard the same stories over and over—the same stories I had experienced my whole life. Listening to these stories out loud, repeatedly, made me realize how wrong I had been about the way I thought about losing weight. All these people spent so many hours at the gym, yet all they could do was complain about how their bodies looked. If they were so obsessed with their bodies and so unsatisfied with how they looked that they were openly sharing their feelings with a stranger, were they *always* thinking negative thoughts about their bodies?

Yes, I realized. They were. And so was I. I realized I needed to change the way I thought. What was the good of spending so much time exercising if I wasn't going to change my mindset and make choices throughout the day that honored my body?

Sitting in the hot tub over those six months gave me a time out every day—a time to actually *think*. I was able to be conscious of why I did things, why I ate things. I had a chance to think about what I did and how I felt. I gained more confidence in myself and in my abilities. And my body started transforming.

Toward the end of those six months, I had a moment that set me over the edge and made me want to tell the world about the secret of my success. I was getting out of the hot tub when an overweight woman who'd just completed two one-hour aerobic classes stopped me to ask where I'd bought my swimsuit. It was a black one-piece, but far from ordinary. While the back was conservative, the front plunged to a low-V neckline with blue trim. It was a cute swimsuit. *I* felt cute in it, a feeling I couldn't remember having before.

I told her where I'd bought it and that there were a lot left if she wanted one. She told me she couldn't wear it because she could never look good in something like that, but that I did because I was "nice and thin."

"How much do you work out?" she asked.

I admitted that I hadn't worked out for six months, that all I'd been doing was sitting in the hot tub. She told me I was lucky. She worked out all the time and never lost any weight at all.

After she left, I thought, *Wait a second, I haven't just been sitting in the hot tub*. I had been changing the way I thought, which changed what I did. I was "nice and thin" because the way I thought about myself and treated myself was, for the first time, truly "nice."

At that moment, I wanted to chase that woman down and tell her that she needed to change her mindset if she, too, wanted to lose weight. I wanted to knock some sense into her. She was *me*, six months before—a woman who instead of being proud of herself for working out for two hours was comparing herself to another person and insulting herself. No wonder she wasn't losing any weight.

Do you ever allow yourself to relax and think about why you think the way you do? When you do relax, are you thinking about your To Do list, insulting yourself, and feeling guilty, or are you dreaming, building yourself up, and considering ways of being good to yourself and your body? Have you ever thought that maybe the way you have been thinking has prevented you from losing weight?

Hot Tub Diet Mindset Change

Even though your life is really busy, take time every day, without distractions, to analyze why you think the way you do about your life, body image, nutrition, and exercising.

2

FUN EXERCISE COUNTS

After the last chapter you might think all I did was hang out in the hot tub and watch the pounds mysteriously melt away. Well, that's kind of true. The pounds *did* start to disappear without much effort. But does that mean I don't believe in exercise anymore? No. I just don't believe in doing exercise I dread.

I used to be so obsessed with and consumed by exercise that in fact I once ran a marathon without training for it. I was dating a man I really liked who was really busy. He would usually have one night free to spend with me every two weeks—until he decided to run the Los Angeles marathon to get in shape. Once he hired a personal trainer to work out with him three days a week, he really didn't have any time for me anymore. Frustrated, I wanted to prove a point. I decided to just show up and run the race. How hard could a marathon possible be?

Huge Mistake. Not long after the race started, a large group of overweight men dressed in Elvis suits passed me by. Throughout the race, I felt so out of shape. When I was finally stumbling toward the finish, a club of seniors from the retirement community passed me, crossing the line before me and destroying any dignity I might have had left.

Instead of feeling great when I finished the marathon, I felt as if my body was going to fall apart. For three days I didn't want to get out of my bed. When I had to eat or use the restroom, I army-crawled around my apartment. I had difficulty walking for weeks. When I think about the marathon, I don't remember proving a point. I remember army crawling on the bathroom floor.

After that, you might think I would have learned a lesson about punishing exercise. But I didn't. A couple of years later, staring at myself in the mirror and completely disgusted with how I looked, I decided to sign up for the Coeur d'Alene Ironman, reasoning that it would *force* me to get into the best shape of my life. (Maybe I could fake my way through running a 26.2-mile race, but even I knew there was no way I could just stumble through an ironman.) I started to work out two to three hours a day to train for the 2.4-mile swim, 112-mile bike ride, and 26.2-mile run. My body felt constantly worn down and I was unhappy since I didn't have time to have any fun, but I pushed through the pain and unhappiness because I thought training for the ironman was finally my answer for how to lose weight.

Then one day I met an older retired gentleman—a funny little man who reminded me a bit of Danny DeVito—on a popular running trail. He asked me if I ran every day. I told him I had to run every day because I was training for an ironman. I thought I was going to impress him when I explained that I worked out two to three hours a day. He gave me a blank stare and started to laugh. Did I really enjoy swimming? he asked. I told him no. Did I really enjoy running? Well, no. Did I at least enjoy biking? Um, no again.

"You're too young to be wasting your time with things you don't enjoy," he told me.

"But I have to lose weight!" I said.

He shook his head as he went back to walking the path leisurely, just enjoying the views, not running, with nothing to prove to anyone.

Did I learn from that exchange at the time? No. Up until the accident I continued to be convinced I had to exercise excessively, like on those TV shows where contestants work out like crazy people because there's a prize at stake for "The Biggest Loser." I was sure that if my workout wasn't painful, I would never lose any weight. Despite this philosophy having *never* helped me lose weight, I didn't think any other way of exercising could work.

At the gym I would spend one to two hours on machines I dreaded, working out next to other mostly overweight people slaving away on the treadmills, almost all of them looking like they wished they were anywhere else. I was paying a lot of money to be surrounded by people that looked miserable.

In the hot tub I started to realize it was no wonder that I dreaded exercising. I was associating exercising with not having any fun and being around miserable people! Even if I were wearing my headphones and doing my own thing, being surrounded by unhappy people and doing something I didn't enjoy wasn't helping me have positive thoughts about exercise. In fact, since I was spending so much time being miserable exercising, I would make it up to myself afterward with food. (Anything I wanted—because it shouldn't "matter" since I was exercising so much, right?) When I realized what I was doing and I looked at the vicious cycle, it was no wonder why I wasn't losing weight. Finally, I started to understand why I'd been gaining weight while exercising two hours a day or while training for an ironman.

I started to research how much exercise is appropriate for the average adult. Most web sites agreed that thirty minutes of exercise five times a week is a good amount—enough to lower my risk for health conditions and prevent the natural loss of muscle mass. You could even benefit from it if you broke up the amount of time into different ten-minute intervals.

I was shocked. I had always worked out way more than that—and for most of my life I had been overweight. There was *no way* that amount of exercise could be all an average adult needed. Could it? That day I sat in the hot tub and really examined the possibility that my approach to losing weight had always been wrong.

Why was I wasting so much time doing something I didn't like? Why would I spend an hour on the treadmill looking at the clock every ten seconds? (Over the course of an hour that meant looking at the clock 360 times!) Why was I torturing myself like this? Why *didn't* I think exercise in moderation could produce the results I wanted? Why the no-pain no-gain mentality?

Three months after the accident, when the doctors cleared me for doing low impact exercise for limited amounts of time, I started going on walks with my kids and doing short stints of water aerobics. After three months of doing limited low impact exercises I felt better and healthier than I had when I was forcing my body to train for an ironman. Since I felt better, I was happier. Since I was happier, I started to create balance in other areas of my life—which in turn helped me lose weight.

Because extreme back pain from the accident forced me to wear flat shoes instead of my usual high heels, I discovered the joys of tennis shoes—which before this I had been embarrassed to wear out in public. I'd thought wearing them unless I was running was tacky and sloppy, and I gravitated toward heels because they were supposed to make you look slimmer. As I slowly healed, I began to realize how much I really enjoyed wearing tennis shoes because I was much more efficient.

I could actually chase my kids and play games with them in the park. I no longer needed to find the closest parking space because wearing comfortable shoes now meant I didn't mind walking. In fact, after wearing tennis shoes on a daily basis, I noticed my feet didn't hurt at all and I started to want to walk everywhere. I recruited my family and friends to walk with me, too. Instead of sitting in a restaurant with my friends doing nothing but eating and complaining about how overweight we were, we now were out walking and talking about things we wanted to *do*.

Walking turned out to be an amazing form of exercise. Not only is it free, but it's social. Liberated from the dreaded machines and from feeling like exercise needed to be excessive, I started to actually *enjoy* it.

Do you have an all-or-nothing mentality when it comes to exercise? Have you ever signed up for an event you didn't want to do just because you thought it would force you to get into shape? Do you let yourself have the time to participate in the physical activities that you enjoy? Do you believe in moderation when it comes to exercise?

Hot Tub Mindset Change

Any form of exercise, even if it's incredibly fun or broken up throughout the day, counts.

3

YOU DESERVE HAPPINESS

Most people's lives are very busy and stressful. Before the accident I felt like I was spending my life going from place to another on autopilot. I did so much and was so crunched for time that I ate junk food because I was so busy and because I "deserved " it. Sometimes I didn't even really like the junk food I was eating—but since I deserved it, why not eat it?

I used to do what many Americans do out of routine: I would start my day off by eating a healthy breakfast and I would feel good about making the right nutritional choices. Then I would go to work, where throughout the day I would make some lousy food choices due to stress or boredom. After picking up my kids from daycare, I'd race to the gym because I felt guilty about those poor choices. At the gym I would put on my headphones and run for a very long time on the treadmill. Usually after burning 500 calories I would start to feel good about myself again. But I would also, of course, be very hungry.

At the end of a very stressful day (and most days were stressful) I would give myself options: I could either make a healthy dinner that I would have to cook and clean up after, or I could just go through the drive-thru and save so much time.

I would have every intention of going home and cooking a nutritious meal, but I was exhausted. Besides, I'd just exercised for an hour or two (so it didn't matter what I ate, right?) For me, it was a simple choice. After all, I deserved not having to cook or do dishes.

One day while I was in the hot tub thinking about this, I started laughing. It dawned on me that although during my excessive workouts I would usually burn about 533 calories on the treadmill, I would then consume about twice as many calories when I ate take-out or fast food. So, by spending hours on the treadmill, I was gaining weight. What makes this situation even sadder was that after I put my kids to bed I would eat snack foods because I felt guilty that I wasn't spending enough time with my kids. (What was I doing instead of spending time with my kids? Working out at the gym.)

Why didn't I think about the craziness of this vicious cycle before? Was it because I was too busy being busy?

After the accident there was a period when I was only able to go on a short walks around the block. By doing this, I ended up spending more time with my children, who came along. Even though I didn't burn as many calories, I looked forward to that special time every evening with my kids. (No treadmill; no dread.) And since I wasn't hanging out at the gym for hours, I now had plenty of extra time to make healthy dinners. After my kids went to bed I didn't feel guilty about not spending enough time with them, so I stopped emotional eating.

Overall the daily change in my routine saved me about an hour and a half of time. My relationship with my kids improved because I was spending quality time with them. And I started losing weight because even though I was burning fewer calories each day, I was also *consuming* far fewer calories a day. I'd changed my mindset about what I deserved. I didn't deserve to get fast food. I deserved to be happy.

I also started to wonder why junk food was the focus of every celebration in my family—and for that matter, the focus of most celebrations, period. Commercials show people experiencing complete bliss when they are eating something they know is bad for them. People feel like they need and deserve to eat chocolate cake on their birthdays. But why? And did we *have to* celebrate this way?

I started thinking about the message my actions were teaching my kids. We celebrated their good grades by going to the ice cream shop. I made them cookies when they felt sad. When we went camping I let them pick out whatever sugary cereal they wanted because it was a special trip. When we were on vacation I would tell them they could eat anything they wanted because it was a vacation. Was I helping my children develop an unhealthy association between junk food and happiness?

I knew I had to change my parenting approach. I didn't want my children to equate food with rewards. I didn't want them to associate food with feelings. I wanted them to think of food as fuel for their bodies.

Do you associate eating certain foods with certain feelings? Do you show others love by giving them unhealthy food? Do you reward yourself with unhealthy food? If you answered yes, does that reward really make you feel happy?

Hot Tub Diet Mindset Change

You do not deserve junk food. You deserve to be happy.

4

CRAZY ADULT FUN

Why does doing something "for fun" make us feel guilty or unproductive? People in corporate America often end up being "forced" to use their vacation time at the end of the year—as if they didn't want to have time off or forgot to use it. We fill our lives with so many commitments that we even forget to have fun, take vacations, or even dream.

I have interviewed many times to be a contestant on game shows, a process that usually takes place in a group with other wannabe contestants. At the start of the interview, a casting director usually asks questions about your hometown, job, and family. Almost everybody always answers these without missing a beat. The next few questions, however, often force people to hesitate or stumble: "What do you like to do for fun?" and "If you won a lot of money, other than responsible things, what would you spend it on?"

I was baffled by how many people didn't know how to answer the first question. Parents would sometimes say something about watching their kids play sports and then trail off, unable to think of anything else. A single person sometimes said he or she liked to go to the movies or out to dinner. Almost everybody answered the second question with practical ways to spend the money even though they were instructed not to.

Alternatively, if I couldn't make a casting call in Los Angeles, a casting director would sometimes call and ask me to make a three-minute video in which I'd look into the camera and talk about what made me unique and why America would want to watch me win a lot of money.

One day after the accident, I was in the hot tub rehearsing those common questions in my head for an upcoming audition. For the first time I realized that all the "for fun" activities I had been telling casting directors about were in fact things I hadn't done for years. Most of the things I said I liked to do I hadn't done since I was right out of college—a time when I was living life and trying so many new things. I had just lost a lot of weight at that time and knew I looked great.

I thought about why I didn't do any of those activities now. Then I thought of the excuses I always gave myself for why I couldn't—all of which boiled down to I didn't have time and having fun wasn't a priority for me. The only reason I hadn't been stumbling when answering the casting director's questions was because I was always prepared with the same answers.

I decided I needed to change the way I thought about fun. Why wasn't having fun and experiencing life a priority? After all, I only had one chance at life.

I immediately got out of the hot tub and made a bucket list. Over the next several months I signed up for my first mud run, an extreme rafting trip, a zip-lining tour and a biking tour down a 14,000 foot mountain.

I shifted my focus from how much I needed to exercise to what I needed to do to physically prepare myself for the next activity I couldn't wait to do.

A side note: though I really do not enjoy running, the mud run was an unforgettable experience that I think every adult should experience at least once. There is nothing like staring at a bunch of adults covered from head to toe with mud and rolling around in it. This event alone will motivate you to get out there and do fun stuff. It's even better if you go with friends that can encourage you and laugh at the same time. I got a serious abdominal workout from laughing so hard!

A couple of days after making my bucket list, I started to think about the answer I always gave to question number two, the one about impractical ways I could spend game show winnings. Until now, I had always made up answers I thought the casting directors wanted to hear. I realized I had become too practical to come up with a *real* answer. I was so busy doing my daily routine that I'd given up dreaming about what I would do for fun if money weren't an issue.

When I finally allowed myself time to really think about what I would do if I won a lot of money, I realized most of what I wanted to do didn't *require* much money, or any at all. So why wasn't I doing what I really wanted to do?

After I started to do things I had always dreamed of, I learned that having regular fun was one of the most productive ways to lose weight.

Are you so weighed down with being responsible that you're forgetting to enjoy your life? Have you ever considered that your weight may be tied to your feeling that you have to be responsible all the time? If you focused on fun and exciting adventures coming up, would you be more excited about doing exercise to prepare yourself for them?

Could you make in audition tape? Is your current life interesting enough to talk about for three minutes? If you watched your own audition tape would you want to cast yourself?

Do you know what you would want to do for fun if money wasn't an obstacle? What activities could you do now without money?

Hot Tub Diet Mindset Change

A responsible person realizes that having fun is essential for a well-balanced life.

5

NO DIESEL IN A FERRARI

I have always entered sweepstakes. While most people were watching television in the evenings, I'd take a few minutes to enter online contests. Once, I even won $10,000 dollars in an online sweepstakes.

One day after the accident I entered a contest to win a brand new Ferrari. I was sitting in the hot tub dreaming about what I would do if I actually won, trying to skip over the logical questions like how I'd ever be able to afford the insurance. Would the taxes be more than the worth of the car I currently drove? Where would I park the car, when my garage was filled with kids' bikes and toys?

I started imagining driving the Ferrari. If I won that car I would treat it like a trophy and take amazing care of it, keeping it in the best condition possible. It would look amazing and last for a very long time.

After spending about a half hour daydreaming as if I had already won the car, I realized something. Why would I treat a brand new Ferrari so much better than I treated myself? Right now, I was treating myself like a garbage truck instead of a Ferrari, eating lots of garbage and treating my body like something worn out and dirty.

I thought of a story my mother-in-law had told me about my husband's teen years, when he put diesel fuel into a pristine 1955 Chevy Bel Air and ruined the engine. If someone put diesel in a Ferrari it would also ruin the engine. If you put normal gasoline into the Ferrari, it would still work, but over time it would not run efficiently. For the Ferrari to operate the best it can, it needs premium gasoline. The same was true for my body.

I wasn't about to spend a lot of money on premium organic food, but I wanted to stop ruining my body by putting processed, sugary junk food in it. If I took the time and made the effort to feed my body properly, it would give me a longer-lasting, smoother ride.

My Ferrari daydreams made me aware of a huge problem in my life. I had been spending so much time taking care of other people or other things I valued that I'd forgotten to take care of myself. There was no good reason I *couldn't* take care of myself—it really wouldn't take that much extra time to add myself into the equation. All it took was changing my mindset, and realizing I'm a Ferrari, not a garbage truck. My life is important too.

Do you treat your body like a Ferrari or a garbage truck?

If you were responsible for making all food choices for someone you cared about, would you feed him or her what you ate today? Would you encourage that person to be a little more physically active? Did you spend more time today caring for a thing—for instance, cleaning your house or washing your car—than you did caring for yourself?

Hot Tub Diet Mindset

Treat yourself just as you would treat people you love or items you value.

6

BEACHES, POOLS AND WATER PARKS

    I used to fear summer. June, July, and August meant barbeques at the beach, pool parties, and the annual church trip to the water park. My whole body would be practically exposed. I thought everyone at those places would see I was a failure in life because I couldn't even manage my own weight. Many times, I made up excuses for why I couldn't go to such places because I was so ashamed of the way I looked in a swimsuit.

    In college I once participated in a beauty pageant on a dare. The pageant included four equal weighted categories: interview, evening gown, talent, and swimsuit. Though I didn't have any stage talent, that wasn't the category that terrified me. Thank goodness it turned out that we only had to wear our swimsuits in front of the judges and do a walk down a makeshift runway in the Alumni house. When we were finished, however, we had to leave through the back door and go around the building to get back to where our clothes were. I'll never forget walking out the back door as all the classes were getting out. I felt as if the whole campus was staring at me. First I froze like a deer in headlights and then I ran. I thought I could never show my face on campus again.

During those months in the hot tub I realized bodies came in all different shapes and sizes, no matter how much some people ate or worked out. I met women who refused to work out at the gym, but ate healthy food and looked fantastic. I met women who worked out every day—yet you couldn't tell. I met a very few women who were trying to gain weight. I met some men who worked out every day, trying unsuccessfully to get rid of their beer guts. (I didn't have the heart to suggest that maybe giving up beer was a simpler solution.)

It amazed me that most people that I met found ways to complain about how they looked in a swimsuit. Beautiful women found ways to pinch nonexistent body fat. Women who had chests I was jealous of said their boobs were too saggy. Men who were hot liked to make faces and talk about their belly fat. Some women pointed out stretch marks you would need a magnifying glass to even see.

I wondered why people did this. As for me, I grew up comparing myself to people in movies and television shows. I realized even the extras at shows set at beaches, pools, and waterparks didn't look like the people you really see at those places.

I also wished, now, that I had Kate Middleton's attitude. I was so inspired by the picture of her in a fashion show at her university, where she looked confident practically wearing nothing in front of fellow students. I decided that from that point forward I would fake confidence until I actually was confident wearing a swimsuit. Instead of running and feeling embarrassed in a swimsuit I wanted to be proud.

Why was it that most people I surveyed while writing this book admitted to being embarrassed to wear a swimsuit in public? If over sixty-eight percent of Americans are overweight or obese, the truth is an overweight person will most likely look like the majority of swim-suited people around her. Why not go out right now, enjoy places where you have to wear a swimsuit and be *active* in them?

I missed opportunities in life because I didn't want to wear a swimsuit, some of which would have probably been therapeutic. Not only would have I had a really fun time and gotten the chance to develop better relationships with friends, but I would have also realized I had nothing to be ashamed about. The after the accident, I went to the local water park in a swimsuit and thought, *Wow I look good! I should go buy a sexy black dress.*

I no longer associated being exposed in a swimsuit to exposing a lack of control in my own life. I realize now that as long as I'm trying my best, eating healthy, and living an active life I should wear my swimsuit with pride and confidence. It doesn't matter what my body shape is today, because my body shape is always changing. Besides, which is more attractive: a beautiful, thin woman slouched over and sucking her stomach in, looking at the ground while trying to hide her body in a towel, or a curvy, vivacious, and confident women who looks you in the eye and smiles? I want to *expose* myself—as a woman who is healthy and has the right mindset about her body.

Does shame and embarrassment of wearing a swimsuit in public motivate or discourage you from losing weight? Are you confident wearing a swimsuit in public? If not, are you missing out on opportunities to experience life?

Hot Tub Diet Mindset Change

Bodies come in all shapes and sizes. You should be confident of your body's shape today while trying your best to be healthy.

7

NO MORE SHOES

A survey I read on the Internet revealed that the average working middle-aged woman owns forty pairs of shoes. And I think I know why.

I used to walk around the mall looking for something cute to wear, browsing all the stores going into the dreaded fitting rooms with armfuls of clothing. Sometimes I would try on so many outfits that the lady patrolling the fitting room would make me try things on in shifts rather than bring them all in at once. Yet after all that, somehow all I ended up buying at the mall was shoes.

I had a limited spending budget for clothing so I told myself my shoe purchases were sensible, wise. I wanted to buy cute clothes, but I always found a reason why nothing looked good on me. However, shoes looked very cute.

At home I never wanted to get dressed up because I didn't have any cute clothes. When I didn't dress up I wore pants with elastic and big baggy sweatshirts. Because elastic stretches, I didn't care what I ate. Sometimes I even wore my husband's clothes because they were really big and baggy.

In the hot tub it dawned on me why I hadn't bought clothes in years and why I made up excuses of why I should just buy shoes. I was unhappy with the way I looked and with what the sizes said on the tags of the clothing that fit me. I had kept thinking I would always lose weight and be happier then with how I would look—so I'd wait until then to buy clothing. But the "then" never came—every month I was unhappy with myself when I looked in the mirror, and every month I didn't lose weight. So I would just buy shoes to make myself happier. At least my feet weren't getting much bigger, so the perfect shoes made my feet look cuter and made me feel temporarily better.

I realized this was backwards thinking. I was actually gaining weight from allowing myself to buy just shoes! I started to change the way I viewed clothing shopping. Maybe if I just bought cute clothes and didn't look at the size on the tag I would feel better about myself. Maybe if I wore pants without elastic, I wouldn't eat as much food. Maybe I would make better choices about the food I was eating if I bought something that was a little form fitting.

Really, why did the number on a size tag matter? After all, in one popular lingerie store I routinely bought my bras in the teenage section because the teen "B-cup" fit me better than the adult

"B" (and for some reason the store didn't make an adult "A").

I thought about my daughter, who will one day be a teenager, and will one day go shopping with me at that store. (I'm all for teenagers having cute underwear, and look forward to buying my daughter cute underwear that hopefully no one except other girls in the locker room will see.) I want my daughter to own clothing that makes her feel good about herself. I also want to teach her that the size on the clothing doesn't matter. In some brands she might be two sizes larger than in another, as different clothing companies base their sizes on what market that they are going after and how well their clothes have sold in the past.

I'm not saying I went out and spent thousands of dollars on clothing right after my hot tub session. But I did allow myself to buy a couple of outfits that made me feel confident, stylish, and sexy right then. Doing so helped me make better food choices, and I ate less. When I actually bought cute clothes that were flattering and a little form fitting, I felt cute. Really, what was the worst thing that could happen if I bought clothes right now instead of waiting to lose weight? Well, I could lose a size and my new clothes would no longer fit. And wait, of course I'd be willing to give up a couple of outfits if I dropped a pants size! I realized I deserved to look in the mirror and feel happy about the way I looked right now, no matter where I was in my weight loss journey.

How many shoes do you own? Do you naturally gravitate toward the shoe or accessory department? When you go to the mall and try things on, are you building yourself up when you look in the mirror or are you tearing yourself apart about all the things you do not like? Do you buy clothing that makes you feel really good about yourself?

Hot Tub Diet Mindset Change

No matter what size you are today, you should still care about yourself enough to dress yourself in a way that makes you feel confident.

8

LATTE PLEASE, BUT I'M BROKE

According to some websites the average American spends $1,100 dollars a year on coffee. I couldn't find a statistic on the Internet about how much the average American spends on fresh fruits and vegetables—but I bet it's less than what's spent on coffee.

I don't want to admit (especially because my husband will be reading this!) how much I used to spend on drinks at the local coffee shop. Let's just say the owner of the store next to my house has probably made enough money off me to retire.

I didn't even really like most of the drinks I would order, but I had to buy something if I wanted to sit there and work on my laptop. This was my routine for years, and I really never thought much about it. The store was crowded and everybody was paying five bucks for a drink—it's what people *did*, I figured.

Later in the day I would go to lunch with coworkers and just get an inexpensive, fatty, fried appetizer. Why? Because everything else was so expensive. The healthy meals cost five dollars more and I was always broke—there was no way I could order one. I could have ordered soup, but that wasn't filling enough, and why pay for a house salad— usually a couple of pieces of lettuce with a tomato on top and maybe some croutons, if you were lucky. I thought buying a house salad at a restaurant just encouraged the restaurant to rip off people more.

I never realized that my spending habits were actually affecting my weight. I was going to the coffee shop every morning because I needed a pick-me-up. I needed a pick-me-up because I was not happy with myself because I had let myself go. Since I spent so much money at the coffee shop, I felt guilty about buying a healthy lunch and would settle instead for something that had a ton of calories—because it was the cheapest thing on the menu and I was broke.

One day in the hot tub I started to wonder why I didn't just stop buying coffee every morning so I could afford the food that I liked and that was so much healthier.

Now I make my own drinks at home, and if I do go out for lunch I'm okay with spending a little extra money on something healthy. In the long run it's actually less expensive, because I don't have to buy bigger clothes. I'm also far more productive at work when I eat healthy food because afterwards I don't feel like a beached whale that needs a nap.

Why is it that a lot of people eat out a lot, but they don't buy fresh fruits and vegetables because they cost too much? How is it that at a restaurant a nine-dollar glass of wine seems normal, but a fruit plate costing that much is way too expensive? Why do people spend so much on coffee in the morning and then go to a fast food restaurant and order the terrible-for-you food off the dollar menu?

Have you thought about why you buy the foods that you do? Is it because they are fast, cheap, and easy, or do you really enjoy eating them? Have you ever sat down and thought about ways you could change your spending to make eating well a priority? Are you willing to stop operating on autopilot and change the way you spend in order to shrink your waistline?

<u>Hot Tub Diet Mindset Change</u>

You need to change the way you value food if you are going to change your waistline.

9

KIDS' MENU AT THE DOOR

The average adult needs between 1,500 and 2,000 calories a day, but many restaurant meals contain more calories than that. One fast food restaurant I like has kids' meals that contain about 600 calories. Mathematically, it makes sense that someone who wants to lose weight or maintain her weight should order from that section of the menu, not the one with the 1,200-calorie meals.

Some restaurants, unfortunately, have age restrictions on the kids' menu. Others offer a kids' menu and a senior citizens menu, but everyone else is left with a choice of meals big enough to feed a village. I used to just accept this fact. If I was in a restaurant and I wasn't that hungry, I would want to order off of the kids menu, but I would be too embarrassed to ask the waiter, especially if I was with coworkers or in a group of people I didn't know. So I would get a normal meal and because I was spending a lot of money on it, I would eat it all to make sure I got my money's worth. I cringed at the thought of wasting food, so there was no way I was leaving food on my plate.

The age-old diet advice of asking the waiter to put half in the box to take home wasn't an option for me. I know some people like leftovers, but I happen to despise them. Maybe it's because when restaurant food cools down, all the grease forms together and forms a thick hard white shell around whatever is left. At least when I was eating the food the first time, I could remain oblivious to how much grease there really was.

In the hot tub I realized that the fact that restaurants had age limits on their menus was absurd. When I walked into a grocery store, I could buy just the amount of food I was going to eat. You can buy just the amount you need of most items— except for toilet paper at a warehouse store. So why couldn't I buy just the amount of food that I was going to eat at that sitting? I wanted to start a restaurant revolution, where every place would serve healthy portions.

But wait, even if I couldn't start a revolution, I could control what I did. If a restaurant wouldn't let me order from the kids' menu, I could just leave and never return. It wasn't my loss—there were at least over a hundred other restaurants in my city and this one would be losing a valuable customer.

From that point on, when wasn't that hungry, I asked waiters if I could order off of the kids' menu, no longer embarrassed or worrying about my coworkers thinking I was high maintenance. About half the waiters said I could. The other half pointed out the age on the menu and looked at me like I was an idiot. Once a waiter asked if I was on a diet. "Yes," I replied, smiling and looking him right in the eyes, "I'm on the hot tub diet."

Now if the restaurant won't let me order from the kids' menu, I'll get up and walk out the door. Depending on how the waiter handled the situation, I might post about it afterwards on my social media page. Speaking up this way, and not being embarrassed to walk out the door, has helped me save myself from many extra pounds of fat.

Some people in the restaurant industry might think this is extreme and unethical. But I think wasting food is unethical. If restaurants want people to stop ordering off of the kids' menu, they should offer the option of smaller meal portions. Not smaller, fried fatty unhealthy appetizers—smaller *meals.*

What do you do when you go out to a restaurant and you're not that hungry? Do you force yourself to eat too much food because you don't want the huge meal to go to waste? Have you ever thought about ordering from the kids' menu or seniors' menu?

Hot Tub Diet Mindset Change

It's okay to order off of the kids' menu. In most restaurants the kids' menu contains the actual portion sizes an average adult needs.

10

BROWN MUSHY BANANAS

If a convenience store offers any kind of healthy food, it's usually brown mushy bananas. To make matters worse, right next to the nasty bananas is an already-hard-to-resist candy bar—on sale.

Like most Americans I'm often at the gas station, whether it's to pay for gas, get quarters for the air machine, buy a lottery ticket, or use the bathroom. Inside the convenience store where you pay for gas when the automatic pay station is down (which seems to happen way too often) are shelves of junk food wrapped in enticing packages that make me want to grab and eat them.

Where I grew up in southern California, most convenience stores would not allow you to use the restroom unless you bought something. Knowing it would take me too much time in traffic to get anywhere else I would just buy something little. I knew I should buy water, but the powdered donuts were staring at me, and I couldn't help myself. Besides why would I pay for water when I could get water so many other places for free?

And then there was the lottery—another reason to visit powdered donut heaven. Like everyone else, I would stop to buy a ticket when the lottery was over 200 million. Not wanting to look like a compulsive gambler standing in line for the lottery, I would grab the donuts again. And when the pay stations outside broke and I had to get gas, I was forced to go inside the store again. The powdered donuts never stopped calling to me.

This habit was at one point so out of control that once, as I paid for a package of those donuts, a boyfriend asked, "Have you ever thought about portion control?" You might think someone you love telling you to eat healthier would encourage you to change. Instead, his question made me furious. I kept wondering how someone who loved me could both try to change my routine and insult me.

In the hot tub I started to consider what was wrong with this picture. Why did I remember him saying "portion control" so vividly? Why *was* I buying an excessive amount of powdered donuts? It wasn't as if I could avoid convenience stores for the entire rest of my life—with three small kids, I was always stopping at gas stations—so I'd have to make some changes in my thinking patterns around them.

I told myself it was okay to just buy water when I stopped, even if I felt like I was getting ripped off. The cost of a bottle of water, after all, was far cheaper than that of a weight loss seminar. I considered that it was okay to buy a lottery ticket now or then without caring about what anyone else is thinking. I realize now that in fact no one in line is evaluating what I'm buying.

I have trained myself to mentally prepare before entering a convenience store. I know ahead of time that I'm going to just buy water or occasionally my favorite chocolate milk and get out of there as fast as possible. Last but not least, I can finally admit to myself that my ex-boyfriend was right and I can finally laugh about it.

After I conquered being mentally prepared for the gas station I started to do the same for parties and holiday dinners. I knew going in what types of foods were going to be there. So instead of making impulse decisions and being swayed by temptations I had a game plan that I could stick to. When I stuck to my game plan I was so proud of myself that I felt so much more confident.

Have you ever thought about what you buy at convenience stores? Do you have a plan before you go in, or do you let yourself wander around aimlessly, being tempted by all the items on the shelves? Do you justify getting junk food because the healthy bananas look so nasty? How many empty calories do you think you're eating over the course of a week at convenience stores?

Hot Tub Diet Mindset Change

If you continue to go to the same place, have a plan in mind before you go. That way, you will be able to make better food choices.

11

THROW AWAY YOUR FOOD JOURNAL

Before the accident I kept a food journal and I was always very disappointed with myself. I'm a bit of a perfectionist, so if it wasn't a good food day I would just want to give up. The more I focused on food, the more I wanted to eat. Every time I would eat something I shouldn't have eaten, I would not only feel guilt over eating it, but I would also feel like I was a failure when I had to write it down.

One day in the hot tub it occurred to me that I should try the same approach to lose weight as I took with my finances—focusing on my daily financial choices and future financial goals instead of bemoaning past mistakes and the fact that I was broke.

Why in my right mind would I want to list everything I ate and then literally carry it around with me? Why review it every night and relive where I fell off the wagon? Why would I want to spend the whole day focused on food? Couldn't I instead just change my mindset and rely on myself throughout the day to make better food choices?

When I tried to assess the reasons I carried around a food journal, I couldn't come up with any good ones. I started to realize that for me only bad things came from the food journal. It wasn't helping me lose weight—it was prohibiting me from losing weight. My entire focus was on what I ate, when I ate, and how many calories I ate. In the evenings I was depressed, since all I could think about was all the bad choices I had made throughout the day. I would feel like I had no willpower and that there wasn't any reason to even *try* to eat healthy or lose weight.

In the hot tub I wondered what might happen if I instead carried around a journal of thoughts, dreams, and goals. The most successful business people I knew were always coming up with new ideas and immediately writing them down. Why waste so much time writing down calories instead of goals?

All day long I would think about what I wanted to do and what I wanted to accomplish. Occasionally I even thought something positive about myself, but since I wasn't taking the time to write it down right away I would always forgetting it.

I decided to change my mindset and I started to carry a thoughts, dreams, and goals journal. I even brought my new journal to Disneyland, where I could come up with ideas while standing in line for Space

Mountain for two hours. In fact, while I was waiting to meet a princess at Disneyland, I wrote down ideas and deadlines for myself in order to accomplish this book! When I stayed focused on the future, I started making better choices, including better food choices.

Why not take the time to write down all the brilliant ideas you think up? At first, taking a journal with you everywhere might feel a little strange. Friends or coworkers might even crack some jokes. (But so what? I was probably the only person at Disneyland with a journal—and doing so helped me write this book.)

At first you might not even have that much to write about, but in time you will. I thought about myself as naturally a happy person with big dreams, so when I first started to keep a journal I was shocked at how much time I spent on negative thoughts about my body and food. In the beginning, the journal was a little empty because I wouldn't allow myself to include those negative thoughts there. After about a month, however, carrying a journal became a habit just like carrying my cell phone, I ended up writing down more, and I was excited to read what I wrote.

Do you have thoughts and dreams that excite you during the day but get lost by evening because you're so busy? Do you write down everything you eat but nothing you wish for? Are you willing to try something new that would take your focus off food and the negative thoughts you have about your body?

Are you ready to take the first step in following your dreams?

Hot Tub Diet Mindset Change

Carry around a thoughts, dreams, and goals journal. Record them immediately and review your journal on a weekly basis.

12

CAN I LIVE WITHOUT IT

It's easier for people with addictions to spend time focusing on other people's addictions instead of their own, wondering, for instance, why anyone would smoke when the cigarette packages themselves say the product can cause death. Often, people who are overweight judge others for unhealthy addictions, yet most people overweight have an unhealthy addiction to food. In my case it was food and diet soda.

I used to be best friends with the workers at the gas station right by my house. I would stop for a forty-four ounce diet soda when I drove anywhere. Some days, I would bring a twelve pack of soda to work. While this is embarrassing to admit (but true), one day work was so stressful that I drank the entire box of diet soda. Since I didn't want my co-workers to know, I threw the cans in different trash receptacles throughout the office. (Can you imagine passing a co-worker's desk and seeing her trash filled to the rim with diet soda cans?) People at worked joked about me always holding a diet soda can, but I don't think anyone knew I couldn't function without it.

I knew all the health consequences of my addiction, but I continued to do it. I knew that I was robbing my bones of calcium and I was putting myself at a higher risk for osteoporosis. I also had already had three root canals and nine crowns. But not even the pain and expense of all that dental work made me want to stop drinking diet soda

You might be thinking an addiction to diet soda isn't a big deal. But the truth is an addiction to anything is a huge deal. Being unable to control one aspect of your life affects how much confidence you have in controlling other areas in your life. *I've already done this bad thing,* the thinking goes, *so I might as well now do this worse one.*

One day when I was soaking in the hot tub and had time to really think, I had some clarity about why I relied on diet soda.

There were so many reasons. Going to the gas station was a quick escape when I didn't want to deal with my current thoughts. When I sat down and drank a soda I could just forget about all the negative thoughts and focus on just drinking. Most importantly, I drank diet soda hoping it would fill me up so I wouldn't eat too much food.

In doing some research, I found out that some studies suggest that diet soda actually makes you crave sweets more. These same studies found that people who were addicted to diet soda weighed more than people who drank regular soda.

What bothered me the most, when I was in the hot tub thinking about my addiction to diet soda, was the realization that I drank diet soda as a way to sabotage myself. I didn't really like running on the treadmills every day at the gym, so by drinking a diet soda on the way there, I could justify only walking. Because I only walked on the treadmills instead of ran I could justify why I didn't look as great as some other people on the machines. And really, since I already didn't look that great, it didn't matter what I ate!

I'd thought I was drinking diet soda to help me lose weight, but the opposite turned out to be true. By drinking diet soda I was, in fact, preventing myself from exercising to my truest potential and I was gaining weight from eating more.

After changing my mindset, and deciding not to drink diet soda constantly, I realized I really did not like the taste. After a couple of days without diet soda, having one made my stomach feel upset. I now wonder how could I have ever sat down and gone through an entire twelve pack during a couple of hours at work. Instead of guzzling diet soda, I now try to work through my thoughts, journaling my positive thoughts instead of just trying to escape reality. As a result I have been able to leave my addiction to diet soda behind, as well as the weight-related excuses I associated with it.

Do you have an addiction to television, surfing the Internet, sleeping, or any other thing? Is that addiction contributing to your food addiction?   Do you ever feel like if you can't control one area of your life you might as well give up controlling your weight? Have you ever sat down and thought about what you do on a daily basis to escape reality when you are stressed?

Hot Tub Diet Mindset Change

You can move past your addiction once you understand why you couldn't give it up in the past and choose to overcome it in the future.

13

NO MORE FAD DIET OF THE WEEK

Search the Internet for fad diets, and you'll find hundreds out there. I think I have tried over half of these crazy ideas to lose weight. Once I tried losing ten pounds in one week by drinking juice and eating cabbage, but really how long is just drinking juice or eating cabbage soup possible? Some of the fad diets go to the extreme of saying you can't eat any fruit. How can that even be healthy? On one fad diet you can eat as much of an ingredient as you want, while the next fad diet tells you to avoid that ingredient altogether or you will never have a chance of losing weight. No wonder fad diets mess with your mind!

At first I would start fad diets gung-ho about the fact that this time I was really going to lose weight. After several days, however, I would start to think the diets were impossible, so I would just give up and feel like a failure. Then I would eat probably as many calories as I lost over the preceding days because I felt so hungry.

In the hot tub I started to consider why I was so excited to jump on the bandwagon of every new fad diet. If every fad diet I had tried in the past had failed my waistline and also made me *feel* like a failure, why would I continue to do this? Why did I waste so much money on books that told me exactly what I had to eat every meal in order to look good? Did I really think I was going to follow the meal plan in one book for the rest of my life? How much of same meal could I possible eat and keep my sanity? Why was I so focused on the new fad, but not the big picture?

I realized that none of these fads were sustainable long term, especially if I wasn't excited about the diet after the third day. So by starting these fad diets I was always setting myself up to be a quitter, making me feel worse about myself and leading to more long-term weight gain. The solution to breaking this cycle was simple: I shouldn't ever undertake fad diets besides they did not work.

Knowing the "secret" to weight loss was eat less and exercise more, I decided to change my mindset and start focusing on that basic principle instead of any new fad diets. That philosophy was definitely sustainable long term. I could follow the "eat less and exercise more" diet if I was on the road, at a party, or at home. I wouldn't have to carry around a book of limiting ingredients or monitor the exact times I had to eat. I could eat anything healthy and not spend so much time focusing on what I *couldn't* eat. The best part was I wouldn't be filling my mind with negative thoughts of being a failure.

How do you feel after quitting a fad diet? Do you make bad decisions that ultimately make you gain more weight after stopping? What do you think would happen to your waistline if you changed your mindset about fad diets? Why even try fad diets when you already know what you should be eating? If you are trying to lose weight to be healthy why would you want to go on a diet that is *unhealthy* in order to lose weight?

Hot Tub Diet Mindset Change

Don't set yourself up for failure. Set yourself up for success.

14

MAGIC PILLS FOR LIFE

Sure, some diet pills have been approved by the Federal Drug Administration and maybe some actually work. But do you really want to put unnecessary chemicals into your body for the rest of your life? If you lose weight on magic pills without changing anything else in your life, what happens when you stop taking them?

I used to be a huge advocate of diet pills. In fact, I started taking diet pills behind my parents' backs when I was sixteen. I even took laxatives before special events. (What could be sexier than running to the bathroom in a formal dress every ten minutes at prom?)

I thought diet pills would fix all my weight problems. Being healthy wasn't a priority for me then, and I wanted a quick solution. The boxes of pills were so enticing, promising miracles in big letters. I never took the time to read the fine print on the bottom that stated all the potential negative health consequences of the pills' "magic." Maybe the companies that manufacture them should put "might cause death or

67

permanent health problems" in that same huge font reserved for "Lose 10 Pounds in 1 Week."

I hated buying them but still I bought them. I knew that several brands I'd taken in the past had been pulled from the shelves after they'd caused deaths. They were unbelievably expensive, too, and I was so ashamed to buy them that at the register I'd make up stories about having to buy them for an imaginary "really overweight" friend. So if I was ashamed of what I was doing, it was costing more than I could afford, and I knew I was taking a health risk with every new pill that came out, why was I taking them?

In the hot tub, I realized this behavior and the thinking that went with it was crazy. It reminded me of a bad cycle that sometimes happened with my lawn. Every spring, my grass looked completely dead. I'd start to give it water, and slowly it would begin to look a little better. Then, if I stopped watering it, it would die completely. The weeds that had taken root when I'd started to water, however, would remain. In the long term, my yard ended up looking worse than when I'd stated.

When I took the "magic" diet pills, they would work at first. Once I would start losing weight, I wouldn't care what I ate. Eventually, I would stop taking the pills for one reason or another but of course I didn't change my eating habits. So in the time period after I stopped taking some new diet pill, I would actually end up weighing more, looking worse, and feeling terrible. I have never put myself through that vicious cycle again.

Do you take or have been tempted to take diet pills for a quick, easy fix? If you do take diet pills, how long do you plan to take them? Have you ever considered how much you spend on diet pills over the course of a year? Do you really think a magic little pill is going to change your weight long term if you do not make any other changes in the way you think?

Hot Tub Diet Mindset Change

There is no quick way to lose weight. You have to change the way you think about food before you can attain long-term, lasting success.

15

THROW AWAY THE KEY

People say the key to a man's heart is through cooking. (To the men reading this, have you ever said that to a woman? If so, please tell me you were not serious.)

When I was single—at a point in my life when my idea of "dinner" was the fast food restaurant's dollar menu—I used to think I was never going to get married, since I do not like to cook. Once I dated a guy who after a couple of months asked me why I had never cooked for him. Immediately I thought of that saying, "The key to a man's heart..." So for our next date I invited him over for dinner. Before he came, I ordered takeout from a famous Italian restaurant that served enormous portions, then brought it home and put it into serving bowls. I even messed it up a little bit to make the idea that I had actually cooked it seem believable.

He was so impressed by my so-called cooking of the delicious, fatty Italian food—that I started using the same tactic in every one of my subsequent relationships—until I met my husband.

When I met my husband I felt such immediate chemistry and a connection to him that I told him on our first date that I didn't cook. I wanted him to know up front in case it was a deal breaker. It wasn't that I didn't know how to cook. Plain and simple, I didn't *enjoy* cooking.

When we were first married, we ended up eating a lot of fast food and both started to gain weight. Tired of fast food, we moved on to fattening takeout meals similar to the ones that I had pretended to cook for boyfriends in the past. When circumstances forced us to cut back financially and we could no longer afford to eat out, I started buying a lot of processed frozen foods that looked like a complete meal. When it came to food, after all, my philosophy was the faster, cheaper, and easier, the better. The way I looked at it, I was still providing my husband with food—a "way to his heart.

After the accident, I started to consider how a couple of generations ago people ate much more basic foods then we do today and were healthier. I thought about how some of my friends identified themselves primarily in terms of the strength of their cooking skills. I also realized that my husband probably hadn't prepared elaborate meals for himself before he'd met me. That's when I decided to throw away "the key."

I told my husband I wanted to eat a simple and clean diet and that I didn't want to serve a large meal for dinner. Cooking wasn't the way *I* show love, I told him, and if cooking was the way to his heart he definitely married the wrong girl. The fewer ingredients that were in the food I was eating, I said, the happier I was.

I also decided to make sure my daughters understood that cooking shouldn't be the key to anyone's heart. The willingness or ability to cook a huge meal isn't what a relationship should be based on.

Do you cook large elaborate meals because that was the way you were raised? Do you enjoy these meals? Do you cook unhealthy food because it is what you think you are supposed to do to please someone else?

Hot Tub Diet Mindset Change

Unless you are a professional cook, create an identity not associated with food.

16

IMPRESS YOURSELF

Have you ever thought you had to lose weight to impress another person? Have you ever tried to lose weight before a big event to impress people you don't even know?

I used to think, *Thank goodness for Facebook.* Why? Because I could keep in touch with everyone from high school without having to go the reunions. Nobody would have to see how much weight I'd gained since high school. Besides didn't people love to make fun of the athletes that used to be super-thin and toned in high school, but were now huge?

It seems to me now that all my life before the accident I was trying to lose weight to impress someone. Even when I was skinny in high school, I was trying to lose weight. I thought if I lost weight I could be a model and then I would be popular. In college I wanted to lose weight so I could wear trendy clothes. I thought if I dressed like everyone else in my sorority, they would vote me president of the house. After college it seemed as if I was always trying to lose weight so I could look beautiful and impress some guy. If a guy didn't like me, I would compare myself to the girl he was interested in and decide it was because she was skinnier than I was. To make myself feel better, I would decide the guy had to be shallow—all he cared about, obviously, was looks, and I had such a better personality.

After I got married, I wanted to lose weight to impress everyone else because I still wanted people to think of me as athletic. Then, after having kids, I wanted to lose weight to prove wrong everyone who had said my body would never look the same. Plus, I'd gotten tired of people saying I looked great for a mom of three. I thought if I lost weight, people would be so impressed they would just say *You look great* without qualifying the statement.

After much thought, I started to consider that trying to lose weight to impress people was actually preventing me from losing weight. I was so consumed by impressing others that when I didn't manage to do so I would feel depressed, make up excuses, and then continue to make bad food choices.

Why had I spent so much time dwelling on this issue of my own creation? Did I really believe that if I just lost weight other people would automatically like me and my life would be so much better?

Would have being a model in high school really made me more popular? How in the world would have wearing the trendy skimpy clothes that were in style my senior year in college turned me into sorority president? When I was single would I really want to date a guy who liked me just because I was skinny? (What if he'd married me and I doubled my size? What would that guy have done when I got pregnant? Would he have left me just because of my weight?) Why did I care about what others—including people who didn't even know my name—thought about my weight? Why was I so focused on impressing other people that I'd never tried to impress myself?

I realized, finally, that losing weight for another person would never be enough reason to keep it off long term. I needed to spend my time instead thinking about ways to make myself a better person— and not just on the outside. I could accomplish so much more in life, feel better, and change my body for the good if I stopped wasting time trying to impress others and started to impress myself. When I started to think this way, my body started changing. And for the first time, I *did* impress myself.

What is your motivation to lose weight? Is it to impress others, or is it because you truly want to be a healthier person?

Hot Tub Diet Mindset Change

The only person you need to impress is yourself.

17

WHAT WORK IS REQUIRED

Have you ever been to a restaurant that lists
the number of calories right next to the menu item?
Some states and cities now legally require this
because legislators think it will help the obesity
problem. But does this really mean that people are
well-informed about what they're ordering?

I never really cared about how many calories a
meal contained if I was in a restaurant. If it had a
healthy ingredient, I assumed that it was healthy. At
my favorite Chinese restaurant, I used to order
chicken lettuce wraps. In fact, if I was doing takeout
and nobody would know, sometimes I would get two
orders of wraps. Patting myself on the back, I'd take
pride in having ordered a very healthy, small
appetizer rather than any of the tasty, high-fat items
on the menu. I was just eating lean meats and
lettuce—or so I thought.

Then one day I was talking to the other women
in the hot tub about my frustration with having so
much trouble losing weight while I was eating such
healthy food. I told them that I was eating a lot of

salads and those chicken lettuce wraps from my favorite restaurant. One of the ladies started to laugh. She used to eat those chicken lettuce wraps all the time, she said, until she got on the Internet and researched how many calories were in them.

That night I went home, did my own research, and found out how many calories my little appetizer contained.   It didn't seem like that many to me—I still wondered why this lady had been laughing. Then it occurred to me to research how many calories I burned in an hour walking on the treadmill. It turned out I would have to spend *two hours* walking on the treadmill to burn off the calories in that little snack. On the days I ate two appetizers, I would have had to walk on the treadmill for four hours to burn off those calories!

I realized just how clueless I had been. I never cared about the number of calories because I never knew how much work was required to burn off those calories. I had grown up misunderstanding how many calories I burned doing various activities. If I had known that every king-size candy bar I ate was going to require running an hour and a half, I don't think I would have eaten quite so many.

I then started to change the way I thought about calories in food. First, I needed to find out how many daily calories my body needed in order to get to my ideal weight. Knowing this number started to help me make better food choices. This doesn't mean I became a person who counts calories. In fact, I believe that counting calories just makes you become obsessed with food, the way keeping a food journal does. It does mean, however, that I now had context for my daily food choices—it helped put what I chose into perspective.

When I ate something healthy that I prepared, I didn't worry about the calories. But, when I went out to restaurants I would do my homework on the Internet beforehand so I was prepared to make a wise food decision. When I thought about eating something unhealthy I started to equate it with how long on the treadmill it would take me to burn it off.

Once I started to think this way I made much better food choices. I started to internalize the idea that when I ate junk food the calories, even on my birthday, wouldn't magically disappear. The only way I could get rid of them was by a lot of extra exercise. Since I knew I didn't like spending extra hours working out and that there were a lot more productive things I could do with my time, it was logical not to make bad food choices. When I started to translate calories into exercise, the pounds started to come off.

If it were up to me, restaurants would list how long an average person would have to walk to burn off the calories in the meal. Would you really want that huge slice of chocolate cake if you knew it was going to take two hours of walking? Most people have no idea of how many calories they burn on an average day, or how many calories they truly need in order to maintain their weight. So in reality, even calorie counts on a menu are probably doing little good.

Do you know how many calories you need to eat each day to lose weight? Do you know how many calories you burn a day exercising? Do you know how many calories were in the last junk food item you ate and how long it would take to burn it off on the treadmill?

Hot Tub Diet Mindset Change

Is the junk food you are about to eat worth the amount of time required to work it off?

18

HEALTHY FOOD IS SUPER FOOD

Every month it seems like a new article appears with a list of super foods that will magically make the pounds melt away. I used to actually believe these articles and go to the supermarket to buy whatever foods were listed, believing that if I just started eating a specific food or replacing a meal with a protein shake, that would be the key to finally losing weight. Sometimes the lists contained foods I hated, yet I would still force myself to eat them. Occasionally I would even chug a protein shake that tasted like sludge. Why? The wrappers promised miracles, as did the Before and After photos. Did I really believe that all those people in the photos were doing was drinking this protein shake, which was transforming their bodies in amazing ways? The worst part was every month the super foods kept changing. When new, "better" protein shakes came out, I would waste a lot of money restocking my pantry.

In the hot tub I started to think reasonably. If these lists kept changing did "super foods" really exist? Wasn't all healthy food super food? I needed to educate myself about overall nutrition.

I decided to avoid reading articles that promised I could lose weight as a result of eating super foods or drinking protein shakes. With that new free time I started to research nutrition. Instead of reading how-to-lose-weight books I started to read scientific books that explained how different foods affected my body and how combinations of foods affected metabolism. I was shocked when I realized that a lot of my beliefs about nutrition were wrong— they had come from advertisements that were trying to sell me something. Over time, as I became fascinated with making good food choices, eating healthy even became a fun challenge.

While I'm not qualified to be a registered dietician, I now feel much more enlightened and empowered when I make food choices. The process of learning about nutrition made me realize that if I wanted my mind and body to work at maximum potential, I needed to make some changes. I deserved to have a great body and to be happy, so I decided I wanted to eat healthy food going forward.

Thank you for buying my book—and for reading it! But I do need to ask—are you spending far more money on weight loss books than you are on books about nutrition? Do you know how different foods affect your overall health?

Hot Tub Diet Mindset Change

All healthy foods are super foods for your body.

19

TOO MANY CUTE PEOPLE

Some people go to the gym looking like they are going out on their first date with the love of their life. (You've seen them, you know who they are.) These are women who touch up their hair before going out on the gym floor, and already-buff men who fake and bake so their arms look more defined when they lift weights while staring at themselves in the mirror.

Over the years I would go to the gym wearing a unisex big baggy cotton shirt and sweatpants. At the gym I was afraid to lift free weights, as most of the time the free weight area was filled of incredibly well defined muscular men with the occasional woman who looked like a supermodel or a bodybuilder. I didn't want to go the classes because I felt that I couldn't keep up and that the other women in the class would laugh at me. I definitely was not getting on the stair stepper, because that would have exposed my backside bouncing around. This is why I walked or ran on the treadmills while wearing my headphones, my security blanket.

After my workout I would sometimes go swimming with my kids. When I had to change into a swimsuit in the locker rooms I was so embarrassed about my body that I would hide in the bathroom stalls and change. Then, when I went into the pool area, I would wrap several towels around me so no one could see my imperfections.

One day in the hot tub, I asked myself why had I been going to the gym and then filling my mind with negative thoughts. Why was I treating myself so poorly? Would I ever let someone else treat me the way I was treating myself?

Why was I limiting myself of what I could do at the gym and not trying new ways to exercise? Why was I so ashamed about the way my body looked while I was at the gym? Why did I continue to get on the treadmills year after year when I wasn't getting the results that I wanted?

I started to realize I should be proud of myself for at least making it to the gym. Sure there were a lot of cute people there, but if I changed the way I thought and actually started trying new things, I could be cute too.

Though I was scared the first time I went to the free weight area, I surprised myself and had a lot of fun. I left my headphones at home so I wouldn't have any temptation to use them, and instead of avoiding the muscular men, supermodel women, and bodybuilders, I tried talking to them, hoping this would make me feel better. Everyone turned out to be very encouraging and offered help if I had any questions about the weights.

Next, I decided to try aerobic classes. Classes had always terrified me, but since they were included in my membership, why not take advantage of them and get my money's worth? Eventually, I tried all the different classes that were offered. Some I really liked and others I decided were not for me. I tried a hip hop class and realized that I didn't even know my hips could move that way anymore. (I decided that hip hop wasn't for me, but for that one class it was highly entertaining to watch a bunch of minivan-driving soccer moms and grandmas shake their booties.) The best part of the class was realizing that, like me, most people didn't know what they were doing. They definitely didn't look sexy and they were tripping over their feet—but they were smiling, having fun, and dripping sweat.

Then even though I always had made fun of yoga, I thought I would give it a chance. I had grown up thinking yoga wasn't really a workout and that since I wasn't flexible there was no reason to try it. After talking to the women in the hot tub and learning what to expect, I decided to try several classes, as I was told that every instructor had a different teaching style. Some of the instructors I didn't care for and some I thought were fabulous. I'll never forget an eighty-something-year-old man in one of my first classes who was way more flexible than I was and who bent in ways I didn't think were possible. In another class, a pregnant woman had far more balance and could hold poses better than I could. In the past I would have just thought negative thoughts about myself and compared myself to them, but with my new way of thinking I told myself that with enough practice I might be that flexible and coordinated someday, too. Also, I learned that the Corpse Pose at the end of the class was beneficial to altering my mindset. I realized in the past I hadn't wanted to lie still because I knew I would just dwell on negative thoughts. Now, however, I began to look forward to yoga classes and to the time I got to be still at the end of every class. I started to really focus on thinking only positive thoughts about my body and my abilities during the quiet time.

When I decided to try a spin class, I fell in love with riding the bike. In the beginning I would sit in the back, listen to the music, and do what I could. Sometimes I even left the class early because I was exhausted. But over time I started to meet other people in the class, people who invited me to participate in outside biking events. One such event was a bike ride by moonlight at midnight. After participating in this event with over five thousand other bikers riding throughout the city in the dark, I was hooked and started to look for other events.

Over the course of time I started to look forward to going to the gym to talk to my new friends. It wasn't a place I dreaded anymore—it was like a social club for me.

I also started to change the way I dressed when I went to the gym. I still do not wear a sports bra with matching leave-nothing-to-the-imagination spandex shorts, but I don't hide under a nasty, baggy T-shirt, either. Having found flattering workout clothes that complimented my body shape, I now do feel like one of those cute people at the gym.

Do you limit yourself from trying new physical activities because of negative self-talk? What is the worst thing that could happen if you tried something new? What is the best thing that could happen if you tried something new? When you do exercise, are you thinking positive thoughts or negative ones?

Hot Tub Diet Mindset Change

Thinking positive thoughts while you are exercising will encourage you to try new ways of exercising that could be the key to long-term, lasting weight loss.

20

COSMETIC SURGERY FIXES WHAT

In my early twenties I was extremely unhappy with the way that I looked. People would tell me that I was beautiful and that I should be a model, but I never believed them. I thought they were just saying it because I was over six feet tall. I would laugh off the statement and tell them that I was too much of an Amazon to be a model. I had a hard time accepting compliments and would always assume they weren't true or that the person complimenting me wanted something from me.

I used to compare myself to models in the magazines, women so pretty that there was no way that I could compete. They had perfect bodies and perfect teeth. One day I saw an advertisement that promised I could have perfect teeth overnight—and that they had credit plans if you were broke. I thought at least perfect teeth would be a step in the right direction. Everything else in my life would start falling into place. I would be so happy and I would almost look like a supermodel. Oh, and maybe having perfect teeth would motivate me to lose weight so I could be just as pretty as those girls in the magazine.

So at a very low point in my life I went to my dentist and told him I wanted perfect teeth. He looked at my teeth and said they looked good and that I didn't need to do anything to them. I left frustrated. I didn't want good teeth—I wanted perfect teeth. The next day at my gym, I looked at a magazine that catered to the wealthy people in my city. There were eight dentists in the magazine that promised perfect smiles. I called the one that had the best looking advertisement and set up a free consultation. I had nothing to lose, I thought.

At the consultation I was basically told I had an ugly smile and that if I ever wanted to fix it I would have to pay over five thousand dollars. The cosmetic dentist made me feel so horrible about myself that I remember thinking I didn't care about how much it cost or the potential risks. I just had to fix my ugly teeth.

I signed the paperwork that day and had cosmetic dental surgery the next week. After the surgery, I remember looking in the mirror at my new smile and thinking that wasn't enough. I was still not happy with the way I looked. Instead of being happy with my new smile I just started to look for other things that I could fix. Staring at myself in the mirror, I would think about what part of my body was ugly and what could I fix overnight.

After the accident, I really started to put my life into perspective. Why didn't I believe the dentist who had told me my teeth already looked great? Why did I only believe someone who criticized me, made me feel terrible, and was trying to sell me something? Was I really so unhappy with myself that I hadn't considered the potential negative consequences of cosmetic surgery? Looking back, I regret having cosmetic work because of all the problems it ended up causing my teeth.

I started to think about my friends who were beyond beautiful yet still had cosmetic procedures done. I had one friend who gave birth to two children naturally and had another child by a cesarean section. She was a size six and looked fantastic. By looking at her you would have never guessed that she had three kids. She was very successful in corporate America, had a great family, and plenty of friends. However, she was not content with her weight after she had her third child. She wanted to be a size four, and was so focused on that number that she was missing out on opportunities around her.

Whenever we would meet up for lunch all she could talk about was her weight. I would tell her she was beautiful, but she didn't believe me. We spent little time discussing all of the wonderful things happening in her life, instead focusing on her unhappiness about her weight and body shape.

After a couple of months of not changing anything in her life, but constantly thinking negative thoughts she wanted a quick fix. She was an executive for her company and had quite a bit of discretionary income. So she decided to get a tummy tuck.

When I saw her after the procedure and asked if she was happy at the results, she told me that she regretted having done it. But a couple of months later she wanted liposuction to go along with the tummy tuck.

I realized I used to think the same way my friend did, believing a quick fix cosmetic procedure would instantly change my life. I thought I would be only happy if I had a specialized doctor "fix" something about me.

After I sustained serious injuries in the car crash, I started to realize that physically nothing was "wrong" with me. I had a great body that was capable of losing weight if I only believed it was achievable. I started to be thankful that I was able to be active. I even learned to look at my incredibly small, saggy chest and laugh. Instead of being unhappy with it, I was proud of it. I thought, *Way to go! The smaller chest you have, the more fat you've lost on top.* I started to think of the sagginess as a proud battle scar from having three babies. Besides why would I want a strange man to cut me open and risk my life, now that I'd finally started to realize how amazing my life was?

If you were told you only had a few months to live, would you still spend time thinking about cosmetic surgery or would you accept your body and start focusing on things that really matter?

Hot Tub Diet Mindset Change

You will be capable of naturally getting a great body when you start developing a healthy body image and believe that the results that you want are achievable.

21

HOLLYWOOD PERCEPTION

I used to think Hollywood needed to start casting more average-size people. And magazines needed to include more fashion spreads that included real-size women.

When I was fifteen I told my mom that I wanted to be a model, so she took me to an agency. The modeling agent said I'd make a good high fashion model—if I lost weight. I was shocked because I thought I was really toned and in great shape from playing varsity sports at my high school. When I then asked what a fashion model did, she told me that their primary job was doing runway shows and introduced me to other girls who were already doing runway. They were so thin that I could see their bones sticking out. One girl told me that if she wasn't that thin, she wouldn't fit into the standard size two to four clothing at the shows, which would keep her from getting booked.

That summer I did everything possible to become a size four so that I could be a runway model. I wasn't thinking about my health or the harmful things that I was doing to my body. I just wanted to be as thin and as successful as all the famous runway models.

At the end of the summer, I was 6'1" and 126 pounds. The modeling agent thought I looked great and I was finally ready to be a runway model. My mother, however, thought I was way too skinny and looked unhealthy. She told me I could no longer model until after I was out of high school. I returned to high school at the end of the summer incredibly skinny and week. I had a very difficult time adjusting to sports. I felt frail and weak, and it took almost the whole entire year to get back to the level of athletic ability I'd attained the previous year.

After I graduated from high school I returned to the agency and told them I was now ready to model. The same agent looked me over and told me that I would make a good plus-size model. I told her I didn't think I was that big. She replied that a plus size model was between a size eight and size twelve. I left the office feeling horrible. From that point on, whenever someone told me I should be a model, I'd think, *Yeah, a fat model.*

One day in the hot tub I started to think about how those experiences changed the way I thought about my body. I begin to think about how much I focused on looking like the women in the magazines. I thought about how much time I spent watching movies thinking I wished I looked like the actresses. I started to wonder why I had spent so much of my life wanting to look like other people.

The average woman was a size fourteen. I was a size twelve. So why was I so hung up on always thinking I was fat? Then I wondered why people in the modeling industry even used the term "plus." Why not divide models into two categories: unhealthy and healthy. If so, I would fall into the healthy women category—which is where I wanted to be.

I did some research on the Internet. I found and watched several videos on the Internet that showed how much some photos were changed before they were used in magazines or on billboards. Sometimes it was hard to tell that it was the same person in the before and after pictures. I was not even looking at real pictures of women. I was trying to compare myself to people so photoshopped that didn't actually exist.

I thought about all the help actresses had getting ready for big events—stylists, manicurists, makeup artist, hair stylists, and assistants. No wonder they looked beautiful on the red carpet. I thought of all of the makeover shows that I had seen on television, where an average looking woman was made to look like she was a beautiful Hollywood actress. Why was I comparing myself to someone who had a crew to make her look perfect? I thought about how felt after getting my hair done at the salon or my makeup done at the counter at the department store. On those days I usually felt great and would take a picture to post on my social media page. If I had that many people helping me I would look beautiful, too.

I decided to focus on taking a little extra time every day so I could help make myself feel beautiful. I set the alarm a little bit earlier to have time to pick out a cute outfit, style my hair, and put on makeup instead of just rolling out of bed and brushing my hair in the car on the way to dropping my kids of at school. After I started to pay more attention to making myself feel more beautiful, I started getting complimented a lot more often. I even started letting myself accept the compliments without making up excuses in my head. This, in turn, started to make me feel better inside, so much so that I wanted to take better care of my body. When I started to put that little bit of extra time into my appearance, I started to lose weight.

I came to realize that while it would be wonderful if magazines and Hollywood changed their standards and featured normal-size women, the truth is that they're already making so much money that they have no reason to fix something that is not—for them—broken. Rather than my expecting those industries to change, it was up to me to start looking internally and figure out how I was going to change my way of thinking. I needed to start making better choices about what magazines I was going to read. I didn't want to bombard myself with images of unhealthy photoshopped girls in glamorous advertisements. I needed to be more aware of my thoughts when I watched movies or saw pictures of famous people. I needed to remember that they, too, are normal-looking people before an army of stylists transform them for movies, special events or appearances.

Do you compare yourself to famous people or models? Does this comparison help you lose weight or make it more difficult? Do you believe you, too, could be beautiful if you made the effort? When was the last time you took the time to do something to your appearance that made you feel beautiful?

Hot Tub Diet Mindset Change

Take a little extra time every day to do something for yourself that makes you feel beautiful.

22

IT'S NOT JUST ABOUT YOU

Have you ever seen a little girl worried about what she was eating because she didn't want to get fat? Have you ever seen a teenage girl refuse to go to a friend's birthday party because she was ashamed of the way she looked in a swimsuit?

After college I started coaching youth sports. Over the years while I was coaching, I heard many young girls talk about their bodies in destructive ways. Some girls spoke as if all their value in life was based upon how their bodies looked. Some were going to extremes to lose weight. I coached several girls that I knew had eating disorders, though they denied it. I tried to tell the girls that they were beautiful and that they shouldn't place so much emphasis on their bodies.   But I wasn't happy with my own body, so how good of a role model could I have really been?

After the accident, I was pondering if I should get back into coaching after I healed from my injuries. I really enjoyed coaching because I wanted to make a difference in girls' lives. I wanted the girls I coached to walk away from the teams with increased confidence and greater self-esteem.

I started to think of all of the girls I'd coached who suffered from poor body images and realized that even though I would say encouraging things to them, I had been unintentionally contributing to their lack of self-esteem. I would tell them not to worry about their bodies, but every now and then I would talk about feeling so fat and bloated that day. I would tell them what matters is on the inside not on the outside, but then they would hear me say, "I look so ugly in that picture." I would tell them not to worry about a pool party, but then I would say I hated to wear swimsuits. Though I'd been trying to help them, my degrading words about myself just cancelled out any inspiration I was trying to impart. Those girls had looked up to me, and I hadn't considered at the time how much of an impact my feelings about my body would have on them. I decided that if I was ever going to get back into coaching, I had to change how I felt about my body.

For the sake of my own two little girls, too, it was time to learn to think and say verbally only positive things about the way I looked. I had to change the way I talked about myself when I dressed. I could no longer make comments about jeans making my butt look big. When I went to a restaurant I had to stop talking about getting fat if I ate dessert. I had to stop pinching every roll on my body and pointing out my cellulite. I had to stop making jokes like, "A, moment on the lips, a lifetime on the hips." I had to stop being self-conscious about wearing a swimsuit.

How did I expect my girls to love their bodies if I was always pointing out the flaws with my own? How did I expect my girls to be confident about how they looked if I was always putting myself down? I needed to start really believing myself what I was verbally telling others. When I started to really make an effort to be careful with my choice of words regarding the way I looked, I didn't feel so discouraged and I started to lose weight.

Do you believe that you have an impact on another person's thinking? Is the way you think and talk about yourself harming or inspiring someone who looks up to you?

Hot Tub Diet Mindset Change

The way you think and talk about yourself influences the body images of those who look up to you.

23

NO LONGER HIGH SCHOOL

Even after I had children I used to obsess about returning to the same size and weight as I was when I graduated high school. I would always get mad when I weighed myself on the scale because I wasn't even close to that weight. For many years, I thought I wouldn't be proud about losing weight until I hit that magical number.

One day in the tub, I started to wonder if the number I wanted to weigh was even healthy for me. On the Internet I discovered that the average woman does not stop growing until her late teens or even into her early twenties. I wasn't even fully-grown in high school, so how could I expect to be the same weight and size now?

I researched weight charts and the body mass index. According to the weight chart there wasn't a magical number. Rather, there was a healthy range of about fifteen pounds. With an estimated three pounds of clothing, I should be between 151 and 165 pounds to be in a healthy range. The lowest number of that range was higher than my high school goal weight. Why was I trying to get to a weight that wasn't even healthy?

Between the weight chart and the body mass index, there was a 50-pound range of healthy weights for someone my size. So why get hung up on a certain number? Why even own a scale to reinforce a number that didn't matter? Even if I achieved a goal number that number would fluctuate all my life.

While I was researching weight I also researched that a woman's body changes after having natural birth. Some web sites said that the hips would always be a little bit wider after birth. Others said that the hips would eventually return to the size they were before pregnancy. Which was true? I realized it didn't matter. All that mattered was that I accepted I was no longer the pant size that I was in high school.

When I freed myself from being a slave to a number on my scale, I started to feel less pressure and enjoy my life more. When I started to enjoy my life I *threw away* the scale because I never again wanted a number to control the way I thought. I realized it was better to always make good food choices than to decide my food choices based on what I weighed that day. Besides I didn't need the scale to see if I was making progress. I could tell by how my clothes fit.

Do you weigh yourself daily? How successful has this approach been for you? Is your final goal for weight loss a set number? Has weighing yourself helped you think encouraging thoughts or negative ones?

Hot Tub Diet Mindset Change

Your goal is not a magical number—it is feeling confident in the way you look and being proud of your body.

24

What Excuse Now

My list of excuses for not being able to lose weight—ones I used endlessly—could fill another entire book. I made up excuses about why my weight wasn't a priority. In the process of making up some excuses, I would sometimes insult other people to make myself feel better. I would make up excuses about why I couldn't lose weight (and started to believe I never could). Then I would make up excuses about why I shouldn't lose weight because of other people. I was the weight loss excuse queen.

After the accident, I spent several days writing down all my excuses and the reasons they were invalid. I soon figured out that the hot tub, in fact, was not the wisest place to do this, as the lists fell into the water and were ruined. But maybe, on the other hand, that was a good thing because I had to write them down twice. The second time, it dawned on me that the way I thought was my problem.

In the past I made up the excuse I was overweight because it wasn't my number one priority. I would make myself feel better by looking at people who were looked wonderful and toned and think they must be really superficial and spend too much time working out. I would think those people must have their priorities messed up. Then I would rationalize that I might be overweight, but at least I had a better life because my priorities were not screwed up.

When I was writing down all the reasons my past excuses were ridiculous, I thought about the order of my priorities. First was my faith, second was my family, and third was myself. I realized if I was really honoring and respecting my faith, I would have been taking better care of the body I had been given. Second, if I really loved my family and I wanted to be around to watch them grow up, I needed to take better care of my body. I had always thought of taking care of my body as low on my priority list, but in reality, it needed to be part of my number one and number two priorities in life.

One of my past excuses was that I was just "big boned." Seeing past that excuse, I realized the size of my bones had nothing to do with whether there was extra fat on my body. Another excuse was that it took too long to see weight-loss results, so it wasn't worth bothering. When I started to think about why this excuse, it didn't make any sense at all! I started to laugh. Why did I think that twelve to sixteen weeks was a long time? Either way, twelve to sixteen weeks were going to go by. So I could either start making better food choices now and see results then or I could just keep on living the way I was living, remaining overweight or even gaining more weight.

Sometimes I used the excuse that I was overweight because it was extremely hard to get rid of fat after having had a baby. This excuse I didn't waste too much time on because it kind of had an expiration date. It's not like I could have used this excuse after my kids turned one.

Most serious excuse, when I was single I would use the excuse that I didn't want to lose weight because I didn't want to risk falling for someone who liked me for superficial reasons. As long as I was overweight, I knew if someone wanted to date me it was because of my personality, not my looks. I'd convinced myself that if I lost weight I would have the same problem as super-wealthy people did, never knowing if someone loved me for who I was or what I had to offer.

Remembering this excuse stirred up a lot of mixed emotions for me as I sat in the hot tub. Had I been preventing myself from losing weight in the past because subconsciously I was afraid to trust my own judgment? I needed to learn how to have more faith in myself and the choices I made. I wish I could have told my single self to trust myself more and not spend so much time making up excuses for why I shouldn't lose weight.

Now, as a married woman, there was another set of excuses I needed to address—I needed to worry less about how my friends would react if I lost weight. In the past I'd thought if I lost weight my heavy friends would be jealous and not want to hang out at the gym or go out. I thought if I told them I was eating healthy and would only get salads when we went out, they wouldn't invite me to dinner anymore. I didn't want my friends to think I thought I was better than they were. I thought it was a lot easier not to offend anyone and just stay overweight.

I realized that this was backwards thinking. If any of my friends were offended that I was trying to eat healthier, would I really want to be friends with them? If any of my friends were putting me down for accomplishing my goal of losing weight, would I really want to be around them? Wasn't a real friend someone who wanted me to be healthy and happy?

Have you ever taken the time to write down all the excuses you have told yourself about why you are overweight? Have you ever played devil's advocate about the validity of those excuses? Do you take accountability for your weight problems or do you blame others? Are you ready to make some changes and see who your real friends are?

<u>Hot Tub Diet Mindset Change</u>

If you are able to think of an excuse for not losing weight, you are capable of thinking of reasons for why that excuse is invalid.

CONCLUSION

Change is good. As painful and long as the recovery was, without that car accident, my life would have remained the same.

While sitting in the hot tub for several months on a daily basis, I learned to stop operating on autopilot. I learned it was okay to just sit there and relax. When I was relaxed I was able to think about what I really wanted and the steps I needed to take to get there. I knew I wanted to lose weight and I finally realized how to change my mindset to accomplish this.

Sitting in the hot tub or a nice warm bath not only helped me lose weight, but also helped me achieve balance and focus in other areas of my life besides weight loss. I realized I was blaming external factors for my not accomplishing what I wanted to do in other areas of my life, though it was really only my own way of thinking that was preventing me from achieving those goals.

Now that you've reached the end of this book, it's time for *you* to sit in a hot tub or a warm bath and really consider why you think the way you do. What one thing about your mindset could you change, for instance, that would forever change the way you view food or exercise?

My goal is for this book to be just the beginning of a change in the way people view diets and losing weight. Instead of people reading about the same ways to lose weight over and over, I hope to see more books where people can be inspired by what worked for others.

If after reading this you want to contribute your hot tub diet mindset story for possible use in a future book, please submit it to www.hotubdiet.com. I'd love to hear it.

Hot Tub Diet Mindset Changes

Even though your life is really busy, take time every day, without distractions, to analyze why you think the way you do about your life, body image, nutrition, and exercising.

Any form of exercise, even if it's incredibly fun or broken up throughout the day, counts.

You do not deserve junk food. You deserve to be happy.

A responsible person realizes that having fun is essential for a well-balanced life.

Treat yourself just as you would treat people you love or items you value.

Bodies come in all shapes and sizes. You should be confident of your body's shape today while trying your best to be healthy.

No matter what size you are today, you should still care about yourself enough to dress yourself in a way that makes you feel confident.

You need to change the way you value food if you are going to change your waistline.

It's okay to order off of the kids' menu. In most restaurants the kids' menu contains the actual portion sizes an average adult needs.

If you continue to go to the same place, have a plan in mind before you go. That way, you will be able to make better food choices.

Carry around a thoughts, dreams, and goals journal. Record them immediately and review your journal on a weekly basis.

You can move past your addiction once you understand why you couldn't give it up in the past and choose to overcome it in the future.

Don't set yourself up for failure. Set yourself up for success.

There is no quick way to lose weight. You have to change the way you think about food before you can attain long-term, lasting success.

Unless you are a professional cook, create an identity not associated with food.

The only person you need to impress is yourself.

Is the junk food you are about to eat worth the amount of time required to work it off?

All healthy foods are super foods for your body.

Thinking positive thoughts while you are exercising will encourage you to try new ways of exercising that could be the key to long-term, lasting weight loss.

You will be capable of naturally getting a great body when you start developing a healthy body image and believe that the results that you want are achievable.

Take a little extra time every day to do something for yourself that makes you feel beautiful.

The way you think and talk about yourself influences the body images of those who look up to you.

Your goal is not a magical number—it is feeling confident in the way you look and being proud of your body.

If you are able to think of an excuse for not losing weight, you are capable of thinking of reasons for why that excuse is invalid.

THE END

Printed in Great Britain
by Amazon